INTRODUCTION

Welcome to the world of the Gout Diet Cookbook, a culinary companion designed to help you navigate the challenges of managing gout through thoughtful and delicious dietary choices. If you or a loved one has experienced the intense pain and discomfort associated with gout, you know firsthand the impact it can have on your daily life. However, fear not, for this cookbook is here to guide you on a journey towards a healthier and happier existence.

Gout, a form of arthritis, can be a daunting condition to tackle. It is characterized by sudden and severe attacks of joint pain, often affecting the big toe, as well as swelling and inflammation. While medications play a crucial role in managing gout, there is growing evidence that dietary modifications can significantly reduce the frequency and severity of gout attacks, offering a complementary approach to your overall treatment plan.

This cookbook is a comprehensive resource, carefully crafted to provide you with an abundance of mouthwatering recipes tailored specifically for individuals with gout. Our aim is to dispel the notion that a gout-friendly diet is restrictive and bland. On the contrary, we believe that embracing a gout diet can be a delightful culinary adventure filled with flavors, colors, and nourishment.

Within these pages, you will find a wealth of recipes that are both enjoyable and aligned with the principles of a gout-friendly diet. Each recipe has been meticulously curated to include ingredients that can help lower uric acid levels and minimize inflammation, while still tantalizing your taste buds. From vibrant salads bursting with antioxidants to savory main courses showcasing lean proteins and wholesome grains, this cookbook offers a diverse range of options to suit various tastes and preferences.

But this cookbook is more than just a collection of recipes. It is a guide, offering you valuable insights into the principles of a gout diet, along with tips for grocery shopping, meal planning, and maintaining a healthy lifestyle. Armed with this knowledge, you will be equipped to make informed choices and take control of your gout management journey.

So, whether you are embarking on a new dietary regimen or looking for fresh inspiration to enhance your existing gout-friendly menu, the Gout Diet Cookbook is here to support you every step of the way. Together, let us explore the realm of delicious and nourishing meals, as we strive to alleviate the burdens of gout and embrace a life filled with flavor, vitality, and well-being.

CHAPTER ONE

Introduction to Gout
What is gout?

Gout is a type of arthritis characterized by sudden and severe attacks of pain, redness, and swelling in the joints. It is caused by the accumulation of urate crystals in the joints and surrounding tissues. Urate crystals form when there is an excessive amount of uric acid in the blood, a condition known as hyperuricemia. The big toe is the most commonly affected joint, but gout can also occur in other joints such as the ankles, knees, wrists, and fingers.

Gout is often described as a form of crystal arthritis because of the urate crystal deposits that cause inflammation and pain. The crystals can trigger an immune response, leading to intense joint pain and swelling. Gout attacks can last for a few days or even weeks, and the pain can be debilitating.

Causes and risk factors

The primary cause of gout is an elevated level of uric acid in the blood, known as hyperuricemia. Uric acid is a natural waste product that is produced when the body breaks down purines, substances found in certain foods and beverages. In a healthy individual, uric acid is dissolved in the blood and excreted through the kidneys. However, in people with gout, there is an imbalance between the production and elimination of uric acid, leading to its buildup in the bloodstream.

Several factors can contribute to the development of hyperuricemia and gout. These include:

- Genetic predisposition: Gout has a strong genetic component, and it tends to run in families. Some people have a genetic variation that affects the way their body processes uric acid, making them more prone to developing gout.
- Diet: Consuming foods high in purines can increase the production of uric acid. Purine-rich foods include organ meats, shellfish, red meat, sugary drinks, and alcohol, particularly beer. Fructose, a type of sugar found in high-fructose corn syrup and sweetened beverages, has also been associated with an increased risk of gout.
- Obesity: Excess weight can contribute to higher levels of uric acid in the blood, as well as decrease the kidney's ability to eliminate uric acid effectively.
- Medications: Certain medications, such as diuretics (used to treat high blood pressure), can interfere with uric acid excretion and increase the risk of gout.
- Medical conditions: Certain health conditions, such as kidney disease, high blood pressure, diabetes, and metabolic syndrome, can increase the likelihood of developing gout.

Understanding gout triggers

Gout attacks can be triggered by various factors. While hyperuricemia is a prerequisite for developing gout, it does not always lead to symptomatic gout attacks. Some common triggers that can precipitate gout include:

- Diet: Consuming purine-rich foods and beverages can increase the risk of a gout attack. It is important for individuals with gout to limit their intake of foods such as organ meats, shellfish, red meat, and sugary drinks. Alcohol, especially beer, is known to be a significant trigger for gout attacks.
- Dehydration: Inadequate fluid intake can contribute to the formation of urate crystals. Staying well-hydrated is essential for preventing gout attacks.
- Trauma or injury: Joint injuries or surgery can sometimes trigger a gout attack in susceptible individuals. It is believed that the trauma causes a release of uric acid crystals from the tissues, leading to an inflammatory response.
- Medications: Certain medications, such as diuretics and low-dose aspirin, can increase uric acid levels and trigger gout attacks. It is important for individuals with gout to discuss their medications with their healthcare provider to determine if any adjustments are necessary.
- Stress and illness: Stressful events and acute illnesses can disrupt the body's normal metabolic processes and increase the likelihood of a gout attack. It is crucial to manage stress and maintain a healthy lifestyle to minimize the risk of gout flare-ups.

Importance of diet in managing gout

Diet plays a crucial role in managing gout and reducing the frequency and severity of gout attacks. Making dietary changes can help control uric acid levels and promote overall joint health. Here are some key points to consider:

- Limit purine-rich foods: Foods high in purines should be consumed in moderation or avoided altogether. These include organ meats (liver, kidney), shellfish (shrimp, lobster, crab), red meat, and certain types of fish (anchovies, sardines). Instead, choose low-purine alternatives such as poultry, tofu, and low-fat dairy products.
- Increase plant-based foods: Fruits, vegetables, whole grains, and legumes are low in purines and can be included in a gout-friendly diet. They also provide essential nutrients, antioxidants, and fiber, which contribute to overall health and help manage weight.
- Stay hydrated: Drinking an adequate amount of water throughout the day helps dilute uric acid and promotes its excretion. Aim for at least 8-10 glasses of water per day, or more if you engage in physical activity or live in a hot climate.
- Limit alcohol consumption: Alcohol, particularly beer, can raise uric acid levels and trigger gout attacks. It is recommended to limit or avoid alcohol altogether if you have gout. If you choose to drink, do so in moderation and opt for lower-purine options like wine or spirits.
- Maintain a healthy weight: Obesity is a risk factor for gout, as it contributes to higher uric acid levels and increases joint stress. Losing weight through a balanced diet and regular exercise can help manage gout and improve overall joint health.
- Consider dietary supplements: Some dietary supplements, such as vitamin C, may help lower uric acid levels. However, it is important to

consult with a healthcare professional before starting any supplements to ensure they are safe and appropriate for you.

By adopting a gout-friendly diet and making lifestyle modifications, individuals with gout can effectively manage their condition and reduce the frequency of painful gout attacks. Working closely with a healthcare provider or registered dietitian can provide personalized guidance and support in managing gout through diet and lifestyle changes.

Gout Diet Basics
The role of purines in gout

Purines are natural compounds found in the cells of all living organisms, including humans. When purines are broken down in the body, uric acid is produced as a byproduct. In individuals with gout, there is a problem with the processing and elimination of uric acid, leading to its accumulation in the bloodstream.

High levels of uric acid in the blood, known as hyperuricemia, can result in the formation of urate crystals. These crystals can deposit in the joints and surrounding tissues, triggering an inflammatory response and causing the characteristic symptoms of gout.

Purine-rich foods contribute to the production of uric acid in the body. When consumed, purines are metabolized into uric acid, increasing the risk of hyperuricemia and gout attacks. Therefore, understanding which foods are high in purines is crucial for managing gout.

Foods to avoid

Individuals with gout should limit or avoid foods that are high in purines. These include:

- Organ meats: Liver, kidney, and other organ meats are extremely high in purines and should be avoided. They include foods like liver pâté, liver sausage, and kidney pie.
- Shellfish: Shellfish such as shrimp, lobster, crab, and mussels are also high in purines and can trigger gout attacks.
- Red meat: Beef, pork, and lamb are moderate to high in purines. While they don't need to be entirely eliminated, they should be consumed in moderation and balanced with other low-purine options.
- Certain types of fish: Some types of fish, such as anchovies, sardines, herring, and mackerel, are high in purines. It's best to limit their consumption or choose lower-purine alternatives like salmon or trout.
- Beer and other alcoholic beverages: Alcohol, particularly beer, is not only high in purines but also interferes with the body's ability to excrete uric acid. It is advisable to limit or avoid alcohol, especially during gout attacks.

Foods to include

While it is important to avoid purine-rich foods, there are plenty of options that can be safely included in a gout-friendly diet. Here are some foods that can be incorporated:

- Low-fat dairy products: Milk, yogurt, and cheese are low in purines and have been associated with a lower risk of gout. Low-fat options are preferred to manage weight and overall health.

- Plant-based proteins: Plant-based proteins such as tofu, tempeh, and legumes (beans, lentils, chickpeas) are excellent alternatives to high-purine animal proteins. They provide essential nutrients and fiber while being low in purines.
- Fruits and vegetables: Most fruits and vegetables are low in purines and should be consumed freely. They provide antioxidants, vitamins, minerals, and fiber, which contribute to overall health.
- Whole grains: Whole grains like brown rice, quinoa, oats, and whole wheat bread are low in purines and can be included in a gout-friendly diet. They also provide fiber and other nutrients.
- Nuts and seeds: Nuts, such as almonds, walnuts, and cashews, and seeds like flaxseeds and chia seeds, are low in purines and offer healthy fats and other beneficial nutrients.

Portion control and moderation

While certain foods are considered low in purines and can be included in a gout-friendly diet, portion control and moderation are still essential. Overeating any food, even low-purine options, can lead to weight gain, which increases the risk of gout attacks.

It is important to be mindful of portion sizes and practice moderation when consuming all types of foods, especially those with moderate purine content. Balancing your plate with a variety of low-purine options, along with appropriate serving sizes, can help maintain a healthy weight and reduce the risk of gout flare-ups.

Hydration and its impact on gout

Proper hydration plays a vital role in managing gout. Drinking an adequate amount of water helps dilute uric acid and supports its excretion through urine. Staying well-hydrated can help prevent urate crystals from forming and reduce the risk of gout attacks.

It is generally recommended to drink at least 8-10 glasses of water per day, or more if you engage in physical activity or live in a hot climate. However, individual hydration needs may vary, so it's important to listen to your body and drink when you feel thirsty.

In addition to water, other hydrating beverages such as herbal tea and infused water can contribute to your daily fluid intake. However, it's important to limit or avoid sugary drinks and alcohol, as they can contribute to weight gain and increase the risk of gout attacks.

Maintaining proper hydration is a simple yet effective strategy in managing gout. It supports overall health and helps keep uric acid levels in check, reducing the frequency and severity of gout flare-ups.

Designing a Gout-Friendly Kitchen
Stocking a gout-friendly pantry

Stocking a gout-friendly pantry is essential for maintaining a healthy diet and managing gout. Here are some items to consider including:

- Whole grains: Opt for whole grain options like brown rice, quinoa, whole wheat pasta, and oats. They are rich in fiber and nutrients while being low in purines.

- Legumes: Keep a variety of legumes such as lentils, beans, and chickpeas in your pantry. They are excellent sources of plant-based protein and can be used in soups, stews, and salads.
- Low-fat dairy: Choose low-fat or fat-free dairy products like milk, yogurt, and cheese. They provide calcium and protein without contributing to excessive purine intake.
- Canned and frozen fruits and vegetables: Stock up on canned or frozen fruits and vegetables without added sugars or sauces. They are convenient and retain their nutritional value, making it easy to incorporate them into meals.
- Nuts and seeds: Keep a selection of unsalted nuts and seeds, such as almonds, walnuts, flaxseeds, and chia seeds. They add texture and flavor to dishes and provide healthy fats.
- Herbs and spices: Flavor your meals with herbs and spices instead of relying on high-sodium seasonings. Options like basil, oregano, turmeric, and cinnamon can add depth and taste to your dishes.
- Healthy oils: Opt for healthy oils like olive oil, avocado oil, or canola oil for cooking and dressing salads. They provide monounsaturated fats that are beneficial for heart health.
- Low-purine protein sources: Stock your pantry with low-purine protein options like tofu, tempeh, and canned tuna or salmon. These can be used as alternatives to higher-purine meats.

Remember to read labels and choose products with minimal additives, preservatives, and added sugars to maintain a healthy and gout-friendly pantry.

Essential kitchen tools for gout-friendly cooking

Equipping your kitchen with the right tools can make gout-friendly cooking easier and more enjoyable. Here are some essential kitchen tools to consider:

- Chef's knife: A sharp, high-quality chef's knife is essential for chopping vegetables, fruits, and other ingredients with precision.
- Cutting board: Invest in a durable cutting board that is easy to clean. Opt for materials like bamboo or plastic, as they are less likely to harbor bacteria.
- Vegetable peeler: A good vegetable peeler allows you to easily peel and prep various fruits and vegetables.
- Salad spinner: A salad spinner is useful for washing and drying lettuce and other leafy greens, ensuring they are clean and ready to use in salads or other dishes.
- Food processor or blender: These versatile appliances can be used to make healthy sauces, dips, and smoothies using gout-friendly ingredients like fruits, vegetables, and low-fat dairy products.
- Non-stick skillet: A non-stick skillet is ideal for cooking low-fat meats, eggs, and vegetables with minimal added oil.
- Steamer basket: A steamer basket is a great tool for cooking vegetables while retaining their nutrients and natural flavors.
- Measuring cups and spoons: Accurate measuring is important for portion control and following recipes. Have a set of measuring cups and spoons on hand.

- Oven or grill: Having access to an oven or grill expands your cooking options, allowing you to bake, roast, or grill gout-friendly meals.
- Storage containers: Invest in a variety of storage containers to store leftovers or pre-portioned meals. This promotes portion control and ensures that you have gout-friendly options readily available.

Understanding food labels and hidden triggers

When managing gout, it's important to understand how to read food labels and be aware of hidden triggers that may contribute to gout attacks. Here are some key points to consider:

- Check purine content: Look for information about purine content on food labels. While it may not be listed directly, you can identify high-purine ingredients such as organ meats, shellfish, or certain fish in the ingredient list.
- Watch out for added sugars: Excessive consumption of added sugars can contribute to weight gain and increase the risk of gout attacks. Pay attention to the sugar content listed on food labels and choose options with minimal added sugars.
- Limit sodium intake: High sodium intake can lead to water retention and increase blood pressure, potentially triggering gout attacks. Read labels for sodium content and opt for low-sodium or no-added-salt options.
- Be aware of hidden triggers: Some foods may not be naturally high in purines but can still trigger

gout attacks in certain individuals. These include processed foods, sugary beverages, and foods high in fructose or high-fructose corn syrup. It's important to be mindful of these potential triggers and limit their consumption.

- Consider individual sensitivities: While certain foods may be generally considered gout-friendly, individuals may have individual sensitivities or triggers. Pay attention to how your body reacts to different foods and make adjustments accordingly.
- Choose fresh and whole foods: Whenever possible, opt for fresh, whole foods that are minimally processed. These foods tend to have simpler ingredient lists and are generally healthier choices for managing gout.

By understanding food labels and being aware of hidden triggers, you can make informed choices and select foods that support your gout management goals. Consulting with a healthcare professional or registered dietitian can provide further guidance and assistance in navigating food labels and identifying potential triggers.

Meal Planning and Shopping Tips
Weekly meal planning for gout management

Effective meal planning is an essential tool for managing gout and maintaining a healthy diet. By planning your meals in advance, you can ensure that you incorporate gout-friendly ingredients and maintain a balanced and nutritious diet. Here are some tips for weekly meal planning:

- Start with a menu template: Create a template for your weekly menu, including breakfast, lunch, dinner, and snacks. This will provide a structure for your meal planning process.
- Incorporate gout-friendly foods: Focus on low-purine ingredients such as fruits, vegetables, whole grains, lean proteins, and low-fat dairy products. Limit or avoid high-purine foods like organ meats, seafood, and certain types of legumes.
- Variety is key: Aim for a variety of colors, flavors, and textures in your meals. This will help you stay motivated and enjoy a diverse range of nutrients.
- Plan for leftovers: Consider cooking larger portions and planning meals that can be repurposed for leftovers. This saves time and ensures you have healthy meals available throughout the week.
- Preparing in advance: Set aside some time each week for meal preparation. Chop vegetables, cook grains, and pre-portion snacks to make mealtime easier and more convenient.
- Balanced meals: Ensure that each meal includes a balance of protein, carbohydrates, and healthy fats. This helps stabilize blood sugar levels and keeps you satisfied.
- Mindful portion sizes: Pay attention to portion sizes, especially when it comes to proteins and grains. Use measuring cups or a food scale to ensure you're consuming appropriate portions.
- Keep it simple: Plan for meals that are simple to prepare, especially on busy days. Quick stir-fries, sheet pan dinners, and one-pot meals can be great

options.

- Consider dietary preferences and restrictions: Take into account any dietary preferences or restrictions when planning meals. Whether you follow a vegetarian, vegan, or gluten-free diet, there are plenty of gout-friendly options available.
- Stay organized: Keep a shopping list and refer to it while planning your meals. This helps ensure that you have all the necessary ingredients on hand and reduces the chances of impulsive purchases.

Smart grocery shopping strategies

Smart grocery shopping is crucial for managing gout and maintaining a healthy diet. By following these strategies, you can make informed choices and stock your pantry with gout-friendly ingredients:

- Plan your meals in advance: Before heading to the grocery store, create a list of the items you need based on your meal plan. This helps you stay focused and reduces the likelihood of impulse purchases.
- Shop the perimeter: The perimeter of the grocery store is typically where you'll find fresh produce, lean proteins, and dairy products. Focus on these areas to prioritize gout-friendly foods.
- Read food labels: Pay attention to the nutritional information on food labels. Look for low-purine options, and be mindful of added sugars, sodium, and unhealthy fats. Choose products with simple, recognizable ingredients.
- Opt for fresh produce: Fill your cart with a variety of fresh fruits and vegetables. These nutrient-

dense foods provide antioxidants and essential vitamins and minerals.

- Choose lean proteins: Look for lean sources of protein such as skinless poultry, fish, beans, lentils, and low-fat dairy products. These options are lower in purines compared to high-purine meats.
- Limit processed foods: Processed foods often contain additives, preservatives, and high levels of sodium. Minimize your consumption of processed snacks, canned soups, and pre-packaged meals.
- Select whole grains: Choose whole grains like quinoa, brown rice, whole wheat bread, and oats. These are better options compared to refined grains as they provide more fiber and nutrients.
- Stay hydrated: Hydration is important for managing gout. Opt for water, herbal teas, or low-sugar beverages instead of sugary drinks and sodas.
- Stock up on gout-friendly pantry staples: Ensure your pantry is stocked with gout-friendly ingredients such as low-purine legumes (like lentils and chickpeas), whole grains, herbs, spices, and low-sodium broths.
- Be mindful of portion sizes: When selecting items like nuts, seeds, and dried fruits, be mindful of portion sizes. While these can be healthy choices, they should be consumed in moderation due to their purine content.

Tips for dining out while managing gout

Dining out can present challenges when you're managing gout, but with some planning and smart choices, you can still enjoy meals outside of your home. Here are some tips for dining out while managing gout:

- Research restaurants in advance: Look up restaurant menus online before deciding where to dine. This allows you to assess the options and choose a place that offers gout-friendly dishes.
- Opt for grilled or roasted proteins: Choose grilled, roasted, or baked lean proteins such as chicken, turkey, or fish. Avoid deep-fried or breaded options that may be higher in purines.
- Request modifications: Don't hesitate to ask for modifications to suit your dietary needs. Requesting grilled instead of fried, steamed instead of sautéed, or dressings and sauces on the side gives you more control over your meal.
- Load up on vegetables: Choose dishes that incorporate a generous portion of vegetables. Salads, vegetable stir-fries, and roasted vegetable sides are excellent choices.
- Be cautious with sauces and dressings: Many sauces and dressings can be high in purines and added sugars. Ask for dressings on the side and opt for simple vinaigrettes or request sauces with low-purine ingredients.
- Watch portion sizes: Restaurants often serve larger portions than necessary. Consider sharing a dish with a dining partner or ask for a to-go container to save leftovers for another meal.
- Minimize alcohol consumption: Alcohol, especially beer and liquor, can trigger gout attacks. Limit your alcohol intake or opt for non-alcoholic beverages, such as water with a slice of lemon or herbal tea.

- Stay hydrated: Drink plenty of water while dining out to stay hydrated and help flush out uric acid from your system. This can help reduce the risk of gout flares.
- Choose whole grains and legumes: Look for dishes that incorporate whole grains or legumes as a source of carbohydrates. These options provide fiber and nutrients while minimizing purine intake.
- Be cautious with high-purine foods: Be mindful of high-purine foods like organ meats, shellfish, and certain types of fish. If you choose to indulge occasionally, do so in moderation and balance it with low-purine choices.

By following these tips, you can make dining out an enjoyable experience while still managing your gout effectively. Remember to listen to your body, make informed choices, and prioritize your overall health and well-being.

Managing Gout with Lifestyle Changes
The importance of regular exercise

Regular exercise is crucial for managing gout and promoting overall health and well-being. Engaging in physical activity offers numerous benefits that can help reduce the frequency and severity of gout attacks. Here are some reasons why regular exercise is important for gout management:

- Weight management: Regular exercise helps maintain a healthy weight or achieve weight loss if necessary. Excess weight is a risk factor for gout, as it can lead to elevated uric acid levels in the body. By engaging in regular physical activity, you can manage your weight and reduce the risk of gout flares.

- Improved joint health: Exercise helps strengthen the muscles around the joints, providing support and stability. This is particularly important for individuals with gout, as joint inflammation and damage are common symptoms. Strengthening exercises, such as resistance training, can improve joint health and reduce the risk of gout-related complications.
- Enhanced circulation: Physical activity improves blood circulation, which promotes the efficient elimination of uric acid from the body. This can help prevent the buildup of uric acid crystals in the joints, reducing the risk of gout attacks.
- Reduced insulin resistance: Regular exercise improves insulin sensitivity and helps regulate blood sugar levels. Insulin resistance is associated with higher uric acid levels, so by improving insulin sensitivity, you may lower the risk of gout.
- Stress reduction: Exercise is a natural stress reliever. It helps release endorphins, which are mood-boosting hormones that promote relaxation and reduce stress. Since stress can trigger gout attacks, incorporating exercise into your routine can help manage stress levels and potentially reduce the frequency of gout flares.
- Enhanced overall health: Exercise has a positive impact on cardiovascular health, bone density, and mental well-being. By engaging in regular physical activity, you can improve your overall health, which is essential for managing chronic

conditions like gout.

Remember to start slowly and gradually increase the intensity and duration of your exercise routine. Consult with your healthcare provider before beginning any new exercise program, especially if you have existing health conditions or concerns.

Stress management and its impact on gout

Stress can have a significant impact on gout and may trigger gout attacks. Managing stress levels is crucial for individuals with gout to help reduce the frequency and severity of flare-ups. Here's how stress management can positively impact gout:

- Decreased inflammation: Chronic stress can contribute to inflammation in the body, including joint inflammation associated with gout. By managing stress levels, you can potentially reduce the inflammatory response and lower the risk of gout attacks.
- Improved immune function: Stress weakens the immune system, making the body more susceptible to infections and inflammatory conditions. Gout is an inflammatory condition, and a compromised immune system may increase the likelihood of gout flares. Effective stress management supports a healthy immune system, reducing the risk of gout.
- Better sleep quality: Stress often disrupts sleep patterns, leading to inadequate rest. Poor sleep has been linked to an increased risk of gout attacks. By implementing stress management techniques, you can improve sleep quality,

promoting better overall health and reducing the likelihood of gout flares.

- Healthy coping mechanisms: Managing stress effectively helps individuals develop healthier coping mechanisms. Instead of turning to high-purine foods or alcohol, which can trigger gout attacks, individuals can adopt stress-reducing activities such as exercise, meditation, deep breathing exercises, or engaging in hobbies they enjoy.
- Overall well-being: Chronic stress can negatively affect mental health and overall well-being. By implementing stress management techniques, individuals can experience improved mental clarity, enhanced mood, and a greater sense of control over their health. This, in turn, can positively impact gout management.

Some effective stress management techniques include regular exercise, practicing mindfulness or meditation, engaging in hobbies or activities that bring joy, seeking social support, and maintaining a healthy work-life balance. It's important to find what works best for you and incorporate stress management strategies into your daily routine.

Getting adequate sleep for gout management

Getting adequate sleep is essential for managing gout effectively. Quality sleep plays a vital role in overall health, including gout prevention and management. Here's why sleep is important and how it can impact gout:

- Uric acid regulation: During deep sleep, the body undergoes important metabolic processes, including the regulation of uric acid levels. Sufficient sleep allows the body to efficiently process and eliminate uric acid, reducing the risk of gout attacks.

- Inflammation reduction: Sleep deprivation can lead to increased inflammation in the body. Since gout is an inflammatory condition, lack of sleep may exacerbate joint inflammation and trigger gout flares. Adequate sleep promotes the reduction of systemic inflammation, supporting gout management.
- Hormonal balance: Sleep deprivation can disrupt hormonal balance, including the hormones involved in appetite regulation and metabolism. Imbalances in these hormones can contribute to weight gain and increased uric acid production, which are risk factors for gout. By prioritizing sleep, you support hormonal equilibrium, reducing the likelihood of gout attacks.
- Pain management: Gout attacks can cause significant pain and discomfort. Quality sleep plays a crucial role in pain management, allowing the body to repair and rejuvenate. By prioritizing sleep, individuals may experience better pain management and improved overall well-being.

To promote better sleep, consider implementing the following strategies:

- Establish a consistent sleep schedule by going to bed and waking up at the same time each day, even on weekends.
- Create a sleep-friendly environment that is dark, quiet, and cool. Use blackout curtains, earplugs, or

- white noise machines if needed.
- Avoid stimulants such as caffeine and nicotine close to bedtime.
- Practice a relaxing bedtime routine, such as reading a book, taking a warm bath, or engaging in deep breathing exercises.
- Limit exposure to electronic devices (e.g., smartphones, tablets, and computers) before bed as the blue light emitted can disrupt sleep patterns.
- Maintain a comfortable mattress and pillow that support proper alignment and reduce discomfort.

By prioritizing sleep and establishing healthy sleep habits, individuals with gout can support their overall health and effectively manage the condition.

Maintaining a healthy weight and its connection to gout

Maintaining a healthy weight is crucial for managing gout effectively. Excess weight is a risk factor for gout as it can lead to elevated uric acid levels in the body. Losing weight or maintaining a healthy weight can significantly reduce the frequency and severity of gout attacks. Here's how weight management is connected to gout:

- Reduced uric acid production: Obesity is associated with increased uric acid production in the body. High levels of uric acid can lead to the formation of uric acid crystals in the joints, triggering gout attacks. By maintaining a healthy weight, you can lower uric acid production and minimize the risk of gout flares.
- Decreased insulin resistance: Obesity and excess weight often contribute to insulin resistance.

Insulin resistance can disrupt uric acid excretion and increase uric acid levels in the body. By maintaining a healthy weight, you improve insulin sensitivity, which can help regulate uric acid levels and reduce the risk of gout attacks.

- Joint stress reduction: Excess weight places additional stress on the joints, especially weight-bearing joints like the knees and ankles. This increased stress can exacerbate joint inflammation and lead to gout flares. By maintaining a healthy weight, you reduce joint stress and minimize the risk of joint-related complications associated with gout.
- Lower systemic inflammation: Obesity is linked to chronic low-grade inflammation throughout the body. Inflammation is a key component of gout, and systemic inflammation can contribute to gout attacks. By maintaining a healthy weight, you reduce inflammation and promote gout management.

To maintain a healthy weight and support gout management, consider the following strategies:

- Follow a balanced and nutritious diet that is low in purines, rich in fruits and vegetables, whole grains, and lean proteins.
- Engage in regular physical activity to support weight management and improve overall health.
- Seek guidance from a healthcare professional or registered dietitian who can provide personalized advice and support.
- Monitor portion sizes and practice mindful eating to avoid overeating.

- Stay hydrated by consuming an adequate amount of water throughout the day.
- Limit the consumption of high-calorie and sugary foods and beverages.
- Incorporate strength training exercises to build muscle and support joint stability.

By maintaining a healthy weight through a combination of a balanced diet and regular exercise, individuals with gout can significantly reduce the frequency and severity of gout attacks while improving their overall health.

Conclusion and Long-Term Management
Recap of gout management through diet

Managing gout through diet is crucial for reducing the frequency and severity of gout attacks. By making mindful food choices, individuals with gout can help control uric acid levels and minimize inflammation. Here's a recap of key dietary strategies for gout management:

- Limit purine-rich foods: Reduce the consumption of high-purine foods such as organ meats, shellfish, red meat, and certain types of fish. These foods contribute to elevated uric acid levels in the body.
- Choose low-purine alternatives: Opt for low-purine protein sources such as poultry, tofu, legumes, and low-fat dairy products. These alternatives provide essential nutrients without increasing uric acid levels.
- Increase plant-based foods: Incorporate a variety of fruits, vegetables, whole grains, and nuts into your diet. These foods are generally low in purines and provide essential vitamins, minerals, and

antioxidants that support overall health.

- Stay hydrated: Drink plenty of water throughout the day to promote proper kidney function and the elimination of uric acid. Aim for at least 8 cups (64 ounces) of water daily.
- Limit alcohol consumption: Alcohol, especially beer, can increase uric acid production and trigger gout attacks. Minimize alcohol intake or avoid it altogether to reduce the risk of flares.
- Moderate portion sizes: Practice portion control to prevent overeating, as excess calorie intake can contribute to weight gain and increased uric acid levels. Be mindful of portion sizes, especially with high-purine foods.
- Maintain a healthy weight: Achieve and maintain a healthy weight through a balanced diet and regular physical activity. Excess weight is associated with higher uric acid levels and an increased risk of gout.
- Avoid sugary drinks and foods: High-sugar beverages and foods can contribute to weight gain and inflammation. Choose water, herbal teas, or low-sugar alternatives instead.
- Limit processed foods: Processed foods often contain additives, preservatives, and high levels of sodium, which can trigger gout attacks. Opt for whole, unprocessed foods whenever possible.
- Consider dietary supplements: Talk to your healthcare provider about potential dietary supplements that may benefit gout management, such as vitamin C, cherry extract, or fish oil. These supplements may have anti-inflammatory properties or help reduce uric acid levels.

Strategies for long-term success

To achieve long-term success in managing gout, it's essential to adopt sustainable lifestyle changes. Here are some strategies to support your journey:

Create a balanced and varied diet: Emphasize a well-rounded diet that includes a wide range of fruits, vegetables, whole grains, lean proteins, and healthy fats. This ensures you get a diverse array of nutrients and minimizes the risk of nutritional deficiencies.

Make gradual changes: Instead of implementing drastic changes overnight, focus on making small, sustainable changes to your eating habits. Gradual adjustments are more likely to be maintained in the long run.

- Seek professional guidance: Consult with a registered dietitian or healthcare provider who specializes in gout management. They can provide personalized recommendations based on your specific needs and help you create a customized meal plan.
- Stay consistent: Consistency is key in managing gout. Stick to your dietary changes and make them a part of your daily routine. Consistency helps maintain stable uric acid levels and reduces the likelihood of gout attacks.
- Incorporate regular physical activity: Regular exercise not only supports weight management but also promotes overall health and well-being. Find activities you enjoy and aim for at least 150 minutes of moderate-intensity exercise per week.
- Manage stress: Stress can trigger gout attacks, so incorporating stress management techniques

such as exercise, meditation, or engaging in hobbies can help minimize its impact.

- Stay informed: Continue educating yourself about gout and its management. Stay up to date with the latest research and recommendations to make informed decisions about your health.

Importance of regular check-ups and medication management

Regular check-ups and proper medication management are essential components of gout management. Here's why they are important:

- Monitoring uric acid levels: Regular check-ups allow your healthcare provider to monitor your uric acid levels and adjust your treatment plan accordingly. This helps ensure that uric acid levels are within the target range, reducing the risk of gout attacks and long-term complications.
- Medication adjustments: Your healthcare provider may prescribe medications to manage gout, such as urate-lowering therapy or anti-inflammatory drugs. Regular check-ups allow for the evaluation of medication effectiveness and potential adjustments to optimize treatment outcomes.
- Preventing complications: Gout is associated with various complications, such as joint damage, tophi (uric acid crystal deposits), and kidney stones. Regular check-ups enable early detection of these complications, allowing for timely intervention and prevention of further damage.
- Lifestyle guidance: During check-ups, your

healthcare provider can offer guidance on lifestyle modifications, including diet and exercise, tailored to your specific needs. They can provide support and address any concerns or challenges you may face in managing gout.

- Addressing comorbidities: Gout often coexists with other health conditions, such as hypertension, diabetes, or kidney disease. Regular check-ups provide an opportunity to assess and manage these comorbidities holistically, ensuring comprehensive care.
- Patient education: Regular check-ups allow for ongoing patient education. Your healthcare provider can provide updated information on gout management, lifestyle recommendations, and answer any questions you may have.

Remember to follow your healthcare provider's recommendations and adhere to prescribed medications. Communicate any changes or concerns regarding your symptoms, lifestyle, or medication use during your check-ups.

In conclusion, regular check-ups and effective medication management, coupled with lifestyle modifications, form a comprehensive approach to gout management. By staying proactive and maintaining open communication with your healthcare provider, you can optimize your gout management plan and work towards long-term success.

CHAPTER TWO

Grilled Chicken Breast with Steamed Vegetables

Description: This flavorful and healthy meal features tender grilled chicken breast paired with a colorful medley of steamed vegetables. It's a light and satisfying dish that provides a balanced combination of lean protein and nutrient-packed veggies.

Ingredients:

- 2 boneless, skinless chicken breasts
- 1 tablespoon olive oil
- Salt and pepper to taste
- 1 cup broccoli florets
- 1 cup cauliflower florets
- 1 cup carrot slices
- 1 cup snap peas
- 1 tablespoon lemon juice

Instructions:

- Preheat the grill to medium-high heat.
- Rub the chicken breasts with olive oil and season with salt and pepper.
- Place the chicken on the grill and cook for about 6-8 minutes per side, or until the internal temperature reaches 165°F (74°C).
- While the chicken is grilling, prepare the steamed vegetables. Fill a pot with water and bring it to a boil.
- Place a steamer basket in the pot and add the broccoli, cauliflower, carrots, and snap peas. Cover

and steam for about 5-7 minutes, or until the vegetables are tender-crisp.

- Remove the vegetables from the steamer basket and toss them with lemon juice.
- Once the chicken is cooked, remove it from the grill and let it rest for a few minutes before slicing.
- Serve the grilled chicken breast with the steamed vegetables on the side.

Nutritional Information:

Calories: 300

Protein: 40g

Carbohydrates: 10g

Fat: 12g

Fiber: 5g

Baked Salmon with Lemon and Dill

Description: This delightful dish showcases succulent baked salmon infused with the vibrant flavors of lemon and dill. It's a nutritious and delicious option that provides heart-healthy omega-3 fatty acids along with a burst of zesty freshness.

Ingredients:

- 2 salmon fillets
- 2 tablespoons fresh lemon juice
- 1 tablespoon olive oil
- Salt and pepper to taste
- 1 tablespoon chopped fresh dill
- Lemon slices for garnish

Instructions:

- Preheat the oven to 375°F (190°C).
- Place the salmon fillets on a baking sheet lined with parchment paper.
- Drizzle the salmon with lemon juice and olive oil. Season with salt, pepper, and chopped dill.
- Bake the salmon for about 12-15 minutes, or until it flakes easily with a fork.
- Remove the salmon from the oven and garnish with lemon slices.
- Serve the baked salmon hot and enjoy!

Nutritional Information:

Calories: 250

Protein: 30g

Carbohydrates: 1g

Fat: 14g

Fiber: 0g

Quinoa Salad with Roasted Vegetables

Description: This vibrant quinoa salad features a delightful blend of fluffy quinoa and roasted vegetables, creating a nutritious and colorful meal. Packed with fiber, protein, and an array of vitamins and minerals, it's a satisfying and wholesome option.

Ingredients:

- 1 cup quinoa
- 2 cups water
- 1 cup cherry tomatoes, halved
- 1 red bell pepper, diced
- 1 zucchini, sliced
- 1 red onion, thinly sliced

- 2 tablespoons olive oil
- Salt and pepper to taste
- 2 tablespoons balsamic vinegar
- 1/4 cup fresh basil leaves, chopped

Instructions:

- Rinse the quinoa under cold water and drain well.
- In a medium saucepan, combine the quinoa and water. Bring to a boil, then reduce the heat and simmer for about 15 minutes, or until the quinoa is tender and the water is absorbed. Remove from heat and let it cool.
- Preheat the oven to 400°F (200°C).
- In a large bowl, toss the cherry tomatoes, red bell pepper, zucchini, and red onion with olive oil. Season with salt and pepper.
- Spread the vegetables on a baking sheet and roast for about 20 minutes, or until they are tender and slightly charred.
- In a separate bowl, whisk together balsamic vinegar and olive oil to make the dressing.
- In a serving bowl, combine the cooked quinoa, roasted vegetables, and fresh basil. Drizzle with the dressing and toss gently to combine.
- Serve the quinoa salad at room temperature or chilled.

Nutritional Information:

Calories: 280

Protein: 8g

Carbohydrates: 45g

Fat: 9g

Fiber: 7g

Turkey Lettuce Wraps with Fresh Herbs

Description: These turkey lettuce wraps are a light and refreshing option, perfect for a quick and nutritious meal. The combination of lean turkey, crunchy vegetables, and fresh herbs creates a flavorful and satisfying dish that is also low in calories.

Ingredients:

- 1 pound ground turkey
- 2 tablespoons soy sauce
- 1 tablespoon sesame oil
- 1 tablespoon fresh lime juice
- 1 teaspoon honey
- 1 teaspoon grated ginger
- 1 clove garlic, minced
- 1 cup shredded carrots
- 1 cup diced cucumber
- 1/4 cup chopped fresh cilantro
- 1/4 cup chopped fresh mint
- 8 large lettuce leaves

Instructions:

- In a large skillet, cook the ground turkey over medium heat until browned and cooked through. Break it up into small crumbles using a spatula.
- In a small bowl, whisk together the soy sauce, sesame oil, lime juice, honey, grated ginger, and minced garlic. Pour the sauce over the cooked turkey in the skillet and stir to combine.
- Add the shredded carrots, diced cucumber, chopped cilantro, and chopped mint to the skillet.

Stir well to incorporate the ingredients and heat through for a few minutes.

- Remove the skillet from heat and let the mixture cool slightly.
- Wash and pat dry the lettuce leaves. Use them as cups to hold the turkey mixture.
- Spoon the turkey mixture onto the lettuce leaves, dividing it equally among them.
- Roll up the lettuce leaves, enclosing the filling, and secure them with toothpicks if needed.
- Serve the turkey lettuce wraps as a light and refreshing meal.

Nutritional Information:

Calories: 180

Protein: 20g

Carbohydrates: 10g

Fat: 7g

Fiber: 2g

Grilled Shrimp Skewers with Zucchini and Bell Peppers

Description: These grilled shrimp skewers are a delicious and healthy option for seafood lovers. Paired with vibrant zucchini and bell peppers, they make a colorful and satisfying meal that's perfect for summer gatherings or a quick weeknight dinner.

Ingredients:

- 1 pound large shrimp, peeled and deveined
- 2 tablespoons olive oil
- 2 cloves garlic, minced

- 1 tablespoon lemon juice
- 1 teaspoon paprika
- Salt and pepper to taste
- 2 zucchini, cut into thick slices
- 1 red bell pepper, cut into chunks
- 1 yellow bell pepper, cut into chunks
- Wooden skewers, soaked in water for 30 minutes

Instructions:

- Preheat the grill to medium-high heat.
- In a bowl, combine the olive oil, minced garlic, lemon juice, paprika, salt, and pepper. Mix well.
- Add the shrimp to the bowl and toss to coat them with the marinade. Let them marinate for about 15 minutes.
- Thread the marinated shrimp, zucchini slices, and bell pepper chunks onto the soaked wooden skewers, alternating between ingredients.
- Place the skewers on the preheated grill and cook for about 2-3 minutes per side, or until the shrimp are pink and cooked through.
- Remove the skewers from the grill and serve them hot.

Nutritional Information:

Calories: 200

Protein: 25g

Carbohydrates: 8g

Fat: 8g

Fiber: 2g

Vegetable Stir-Fry with Tofu

Description: This vegetable stir-fry with tofu is a flavorful and nutritious vegan dish that is quick and easy to prepare. Packed with colorful veggies and protein-rich tofu, it's a satisfying option for a wholesome meal.

Ingredients:

- 1 block firm tofu, drained and cut into cubes
- 2 tablespoons soy sauce
- 1 tablespoon sesame oil
- 1 tablespoon cornstarch
- 2 tablespoons vegetable oil
- 1 onion, thinly sliced
- 2 cloves garlic, minced
- 1 red bell pepper, sliced
- 1 yellow bell pepper, sliced
- 1 cup sliced mushrooms
- 1 cup broccoli florets
- 1 cup snow peas
- Salt and pepper to taste
- Cooked rice or noodles, for serving (optional)

Instructions:

- In a bowl, combine the soy sauce, sesame oil, and cornstarch. Add the tofu cubes and gently toss to coat them with the sauce. Let them marinate for about 10 minutes.
- Heat the vegetable oil in a large skillet or wok over medium-high heat.
- Add the marinated tofu cubes to the skillet and cook until they are golden brown and crispy on all sides. Remove the tofu from the skillet and set aside.
- In the same skillet, add the sliced onion and minced garlic. Sauté for a few minutes until they

are fragrant and slightly softened.

- Add the sliced bell peppers, mushrooms, broccoli florets, and snow peas to the skillet. Stir-fry for about 5-7 minutes, or until the vegetables are tender-crisp.
- Return the cooked tofu to the skillet and toss everything together.
- Season with salt and pepper to taste.
- Serve the vegetable stir-fry as is or over cooked rice or noodles for a complete meal.

Nutritional Information:

Calories: 250

Protein: 15g

Carbohydrates: 15g

Fat: 15g

Fiber: 5g

Grilled Steak with Roasted Asparagus

Description: This grilled steak with roasted asparagus is a classic and satisfying meal that showcases juicy and flavorful steak paired with tender and flavorful asparagus. It's a hearty dish that's perfect for meat lovers.

Ingredients:

- 2 beef steak cuts (such as ribeye or sirloin)
- 2 tablespoons olive oil
- Salt and pepper to taste
- 1 bunch asparagus, woody ends trimmed
- 2 tablespoons balsamic vinegar
- 1 tablespoon honey
- 2 cloves garlic, minced

Instructions:

- Preheat the grill to medium-high heat.
- Rub the steaks with olive oil and season with salt and pepper.
- Place the steaks on the grill and cook for about 4-5 minutes per side for medium-rare, or adjust the cooking time according to your desired doneness.
- While the steaks are grilling, preheat the oven to 400°F (200°C).
- In a small bowl, whisk together the balsamic vinegar, honey, minced garlic, salt, and pepper.
- Place the trimmed asparagus on a baking sheet and drizzle the balsamic mixture over them. Toss to coat.
- Roast the asparagus in the preheated oven for about 10-12 minutes, or until they are tender and slightly caramelized.
- Remove the steaks from the grill and let them rest for a few minutes before slicing.
- Serve the grilled steak with the roasted asparagus on the side.

Nutritional Information:

Calories: 400

Protein: 35g

Carbohydrates: 10g

Fat: 25g

Fiber: 4g

Lentil Soup with Spinach and Carrots

Description: This hearty lentil soup is packed with

nutritious ingredients like lentils, spinach, and carrots. It's a comforting and satisfying soup that's perfect for cooler days or when you're in need of a wholesome and flavorful meal.

Ingredients:

- 1 cup dried lentils, rinsed and drained
- 1 tablespoon olive oil
- 1 onion, diced
- 2 cloves garlic, minced
- 2 carrots, diced
- 4 cups vegetable broth
- 1 bay leaf
- 1 teaspoon dried thyme
- 1 teaspoon paprika
- Salt and pepper to taste
- 2 cups fresh spinach leaves, chopped
- Lemon wedges for serving (optional)

Instructions:

- Heat the olive oil in a large pot or Dutch oven over medium heat.
- Add the diced onion, minced garlic, and diced carrots to the pot. Sauté for a few minutes until the vegetables are slightly softened.
- Add the rinsed lentils, vegetable broth, bay leaf, dried thyme, and paprika to the pot. Season with salt and pepper.
- Bring the soup to a boil, then reduce the heat to low and simmer for about 30-35 minutes, or until the lentils are tender.
- Stir in the chopped spinach leaves and simmer for an additional 5 minutes, or until the spinach wilts.

- Remove the bay leaf from the soup.
- Serve the lentil soup hot with a squeeze of fresh lemon juice, if desired.

Nutritional Information:

Calories: 200

Protein: 12g

Carbohydrates: 35g

Fat: 3g

Fiber: 12g

Spinach and Feta Stuffed Chicken Breast

Description: This delightful dish features tender chicken breast stuffed with a savory mixture of spinach and feta cheese. The combination of flavors creates a delicious and satisfying meal that is both impressive and easy to prepare.

Ingredients:

- 2 boneless, skinless chicken breasts
- 2 cups fresh spinach leaves
- 1/2 cup crumbled feta cheese
- 2 cloves garlic, minced
- 1 tablespoon olive oil
- Salt and pepper to taste

Instructions:

- Preheat the oven to 375°F (190°C).
- Slice each chicken breast horizontally, being careful not to cut all the way through. Open the chicken breasts like a book.
- In a skillet, heat the olive oil over medium heat. Add the minced garlic and sauté for about 1

minute until fragrant.

- Add the fresh spinach leaves to the skillet and cook until wilted.
- Remove the skillet from heat and let the spinach cool slightly.
- In a bowl, combine the cooked spinach and crumbled feta cheese. Season with salt and pepper to taste.
- Spoon the spinach and feta mixture onto one side of each opened chicken breast.
- Fold the other side of the chicken breast over the filling, creating a stuffed chicken breast.
- Secure the edges with toothpicks, if needed.
- Place the stuffed chicken breasts in a baking dish and season with salt and pepper.
- Bake in the preheated oven for about 25-30 minutes, or until the chicken is cooked through and no longer pink in the center.
- Remove the toothpicks, slice the stuffed chicken breasts, and serve.

Nutritional Information:

Calories: 300

Protein: 40g

Carbohydrates: 5g

Fat: 12g

Fiber: 2g

Roasted Portobello Mushroom Burger with Avocado

Description: This vegetarian burger features a hearty and flavorful roasted Portobello mushroom cap served on a bun and topped with creamy avocado. It's a satisfying and delicious option for those looking for a meatless alternative.

Ingredients:

- 4 large Portobello mushroom caps
- 2 tablespoons balsamic vinegar
- 2 tablespoons olive oil
- 2 cloves garlic, minced
- Salt and pepper to taste
- 4 burger buns
- 1 ripe avocado, sliced
- Lettuce, tomato slices, and other desired toppings

Instructions:

- Preheat the oven to 400°F (200°C).
- In a small bowl, whisk together the balsamic vinegar, olive oil, minced garlic, salt, and pepper.
- Clean the Portobello mushroom caps and remove the stems.
- Place the mushroom caps in a baking dish and brush them with the balsamic mixture, making sure to coat both sides.
- Roast the mushroom caps in the preheated oven for about 15-20 minutes, or until they are tender and slightly caramelized.
- While the mushrooms are roasting, prepare the burger buns and toppings.
- Toast the burger buns, if desired.
- Once the mushrooms are done, assemble the burgers by placing a roasted mushroom cap on the bottom half of each bun.
- Top the mushrooms with avocado slices, lettuce, tomato slices, and any other desired toppings.

- Place the top half of the bun on the toppings and serve the roasted Portobello mushroom burger.

Nutritional Information:

Calories: 250

Protein: 5g

Carbohydrates: 30g

Fat: 12g

Fiber: 6g

Baked Cod with Herbed Couscous

Description: This flavorful dish features tender baked cod fillets served over a bed of aromatic herbed couscous. It's a light and satisfying meal that showcases the delicate flavor of the fish and the fragrant blend of herbs.

Ingredients:

- 4 cod fillets
- 2 tablespoons olive oil
- 1 tablespoon lemon juice
- 1 teaspoon dried dill
- 1 teaspoon dried parsley
- Salt and pepper to taste
- 1 cup couscous
- 1 1/4 cups vegetable broth or water
- 2 tablespoons chopped fresh parsley
- Lemon wedges for serving (optional)

Instructions:

- Preheat the oven to 400°F (200°C).
- Place the cod fillets in a baking dish.
- In a small bowl, whisk together the olive oil, lemon juice, dried dill, dried parsley, salt, and

- pepper.
- Pour the mixture over the cod fillets, coating them evenly.
- Bake the cod in the preheated oven for about 12-15 minutes, or until the fish is opaque and flakes easily with a fork.
- While the cod is baking, prepare the herbed couscous.
- In a saucepan, bring the vegetable broth or water to a boil.
- Stir in the couscous, cover the saucepan, and remove it from heat.
- Let the couscous sit for about 5 minutes to absorb the liquid.
- Fluff the couscous with a fork and stir in the chopped fresh parsley.
- Serve the baked cod fillets over a bed of herbed couscous.
- Garnish with lemon wedges, if desired.

Nutritional Information:

Calories: 300

Protein: 30g

Carbohydrates: 30g

Fat: 8g

Fiber: 3g

Greek Salad with Grilled Chicken

Description: This vibrant and refreshing Greek salad is a medley of fresh vegetables, tangy feta cheese, and grilled chicken. It's a light and healthy meal that is bursting with flavors and textures.

Ingredients:

- 2 boneless, skinless chicken breasts
- 2 tablespoons olive oil
- 1 tablespoon lemon juice
- 2 cloves garlic, minced
- 1 teaspoon dried oregano
- Salt and pepper to taste
- 4 cups mixed salad greens
- 1 cucumber, diced
- 1 cup cherry tomatoes, halved
- 1/2 red onion, thinly sliced
- 1/2 cup Kalamata olives, pitted
- 1/2 cup crumbled feta cheese
- Greek salad dressing, to taste

Instructions:

- Preheat the grill to medium-high heat.
- In a bowl, whisk together the olive oil, lemon juice, minced garlic, dried oregano, salt, and pepper.
- Place the chicken breasts in the marinade and let them marinate for about 15-30 minutes.
- Grill the chicken breasts for about 6-8 minutes per side, or until they are cooked through and reach an internal temperature of 165°F (74°C).
- Remove the chicken from the grill and let it rest for a few minutes before slicing.
- In a large salad bowl, combine the mixed salad greens, diced cucumber, cherry tomatoes, sliced red onion, Kalamata olives, and crumbled feta cheese.
- Add the sliced grilled chicken on top of the salad.
- Drizzle the Greek salad dressing over the salad, to taste.

- Toss the salad gently to coat the ingredients with the dressing.
- Serve the Greek salad with grilled chicken as a refreshing and nutritious meal.

Nutritional Information:

Calories: 350

Protein: 30g

Carbohydrates: 15g

Fat: 18g

Fiber: 5g

Eggplant Parmesan with Whole Wheat Pasta

Description: This vegetarian dish features layers of breaded and baked eggplant slices smothered in rich tomato sauce and melted cheese. Served with whole wheat pasta, it's a wholesome and flavorful meal that will satisfy your cravings for comfort food.

Ingredients:

1 large eggplant, sliced into 1/2-inch rounds

- 1 cup whole wheat breadcrumbs
- 1/2 cup grated Parmesan cheese
- 2 eggs, beaten
- 2 cups marinara sauce
- 1 cup shredded mozzarella cheese
- Fresh basil leaves for garnish (optional)
- 8 ounces whole wheat pasta of your choice

Instructions:

- Preheat the oven to 400°F (200°C).
- Prepare a baking sheet and lightly grease it.

- In a shallow dish, combine the whole wheat breadcrumbs and grated Parmesan cheese.
- Dip each eggplant slice into the beaten eggs, then coat it with the breadcrumb mixture.
- Place the breaded eggplant slices on the prepared baking sheet.
- Bake the eggplant slices in the preheated oven for about 15-20 minutes, or until they are golden brown and crispy.
- While the eggplant is baking, cook the whole wheat pasta according to the package instructions until al dente. Drain and set aside.
- In a saucepan, heat the marinara sauce over medium heat until warmed through.
- Remove the eggplant slices from the oven and reduce the oven temperature to 350°F (175°C).
- Spread a thin layer of marinara sauce in the bottom of a baking dish.
- Arrange a layer of the baked eggplant slices on top of the sauce.
- Sprinkle a portion of shredded mozzarella cheese over the eggplant.
- Repeat the layers of sauce, eggplant, and cheese until all the ingredients are used, ending with a layer of sauce and cheese on top.
- Bake the eggplant Parmesan in the 350°F (175°C) oven for about 20-25 minutes, or until the cheese is melted and bubbly.
- Serve the eggplant Parmesan with a side of whole wheat pasta and garnish with fresh basil leaves, if desired.

Nutritional Information:

Calories: 400

Protein: 20g

Carbohydrates: 60g

Fat: 10g

Fiber: 10g

Turkey Chili with Kidney Beans and Bell Peppers

Description: This hearty and flavorful turkey chili is packed with lean ground turkey, kidney beans, and colorful bell peppers. It's a nutritious and satisfying meal that will warm you up on chilly days.

Ingredients:

- 1 tablespoon olive oil
- 1 onion, diced
- 2 cloves garlic, minced
- 1 pound ground turkey
- 1 red bell pepper, diced
- 1 green bell pepper, diced
- 1 can (15 ounces) kidney beans, drained and rinsed
- 1 can (14.5 ounces) diced tomatoes
- 2 tablespoons chili powder
- 1 teaspoon cumin
- 1 teaspoon paprika
- Salt and pepper to taste
- Optional toppings: shredded cheese, chopped cilantro, sliced green onions, sour cream

Instructions:

- Heat the olive oil in a large pot or Dutch oven over

medium heat.

- Add the diced onion and minced garlic to the pot. Sauté until the onion is translucent and fragrant.
- Add the ground turkey to the pot and cook, breaking it up with a spoon, until it is browned and cooked through.
- Stir in the diced bell peppers and cook for a few minutes until they begin to soften.
- Add the kidney beans, diced tomatoes, chili powder, cumin, paprika, salt, and pepper to the pot. Stir well to combine.
- Bring the chili to a simmer, then reduce the heat to low and let it cook for about 30 minutes to allow the flavors to meld together.
- Taste and adjust the seasoning if needed.
- Serve the turkey chili hot, garnished with your choice of toppings such as shredded cheese, chopped cilantro, sliced green onions, or sour cream.

Nutritional Information:

Calories: 350

Protein: 30g

Carbohydrates: 25g

Fat: 15g

Fiber: 8g

Quinoa Stuffed Bell Peppers

Description: These colorful and nutritious bell peppers are stuffed with a delicious mixture of quinoa, vegetables, and cheese. They make for an impressive and satisfying vegetarian main dish that is as visually appealing as it is tasty.

Ingredients:

- 4 bell peppers (any color), tops removed and seeds removed
- 1 cup quinoa, rinsed
- 2 cups vegetable broth or water
- 1 tablespoon olive oil
- 1 onion, diced
- 2 cloves garlic, minced
- 1 zucchini, diced
- 1 carrot, diced
- 1 cup diced tomatoes
- 1 teaspoon dried oregano
- 1 teaspoon dried basil
- Salt and pepper to taste
- 1 cup shredded mozzarella cheese

Instructions:

- Preheat the oven to 375°F (190°C).
- In a saucepan, bring the vegetable broth or water to a boil.
- Add the rinsed quinoa to the boiling liquid, cover the saucepan, and reduce the heat to low.
- Simmer the quinoa for about 15 minutes, or until all the liquid is absorbed and the quinoa is cooked.
- In a separate skillet, heat the olive oil over medium heat.
- Add the diced onion and minced garlic to the skillet. Sauté until the onion is translucent and fragrant.
- Add the diced zucchini and carrot to the skillet and cook for a few minutes until they begin to soften.

- Stir in the diced tomatoes, dried oregano, dried basil, salt, and pepper. Cook for another few minutes to allow the flavors to meld together.
- In a large mixing bowl, combine the cooked quinoa and the vegetable mixture.
- Stir in the shredded mozzarella cheese and mix until well combined.
- Stuff the bell peppers with the quinoa mixture, pressing it down gently to fill the peppers.
- Place the stuffed bell peppers in a baking dish and cover the dish with foil.
- Bake in the preheated oven for about 25-30 minutes, or until the bell peppers are tender.
- Remove the foil and bake for an additional 5 minutes to allow the cheese to melt and lightly brown.
- Serve the quinoa stuffed bell peppers as a delicious and satisfying vegetarian main dish.

Nutritional Information:

Calories: 300

Protein: 12g

Carbohydrates: 45g

Fat: 8g

Fiber: 8g

Grilled Halibut with Mango Salsa

Description: This light and flavorful dish features tender grilled halibut fillets topped with a vibrant and refreshing mango salsa. It's a perfect combination of juicy seafood and tropical flavors that will transport you to a sunny paradise.

Ingredients:

- 2 halibut fillets
- 2 tablespoons olive oil
- 1 tablespoon lemon juice
- 1 teaspoon dried thyme
- Salt and pepper to taste
- 1 ripe mango, peeled and diced
- 1/2 red bell pepper, diced
- 1/2 red onion, diced
- 1 jalapeño pepper, seeded and finely chopped
- 2 tablespoons chopped fresh cilantro
- 1 tablespoon lime juice

Instructions:

- Preheat the grill to medium-high heat.
- In a small bowl, whisk together the olive oil, lemon juice, dried thyme, salt, and pepper.
- Brush the halibut fillets with the prepared marinade, coating them evenly.
- Grill the halibut fillets for about 4-5 minutes per side, or until they are cooked through and flake easily with a fork.
- While the halibut is grilling, prepare the mango salsa.
- In a mixing bowl, combine the diced mango, diced red bell pepper, diced red onion, chopped jalapeño pepper, chopped fresh cilantro, and lime juice.
- Toss the ingredients together until well mixed.
- Remove the grilled halibut from the heat and let it rest for a few minutes.
- Serve the halibut fillets hot, topped with the refreshing mango salsa.

Nutritional Information:

Calories: 300

Protein: 30g

Carbohydrates: 15g

Fat: 12g

Fiber: 3g

CONCLUSION

In conclusion, the Gout Diet Cookbook serves as an invaluable resource for individuals seeking to manage and alleviate the symptoms of gout through dietary modifications. By providing a comprehensive collection of delicious recipes, helpful tips, and nutritional guidance, this cookbook empowers readers to make informed choices that support their overall health and well-being. Through the incorporation of gout-friendly ingredients and mindful meal planning, individuals can regain control over their diet, reduce the frequency of painful gout attacks, and enhance their quality of life. Embracing this cookbook as a guide on their journey towards better health, readers will discover a newfound sense of culinary enjoyment and personal empowerment, paving the way for a happier, more vibrant life free from the constraints of gout.